Homemade Painkillers

Natural Creams, Sprays, and Tea Herbs for Pain Relief

Table of Contents

Introduction

This world we live in is full of modern day advantages that those who lived before never got to enjoy. Now, when you are sick, you go to the doctor, you are given some medication, and you come home. Problem solved.

Or so we think.

In this modern world, we are taught to believe that all our problems can be solved with pills. Anything and everything that bothers you can be fixed with nothing more than a little pill administered a couple times per day. At first, it might not sound like a bad idea.

But then you realize that there are side effects. Though these pills are designed to get rid of a number of symptoms, what they don't tell you is that these pills also bring with them side effects that can be even more harmful to the body than the aches and pains you were feeling in the first place.

Of course, this doesn't mean that you have to live with your pain. In fact, there is a reason people have chosen to use herbal remedies for thousands of years. It's because they work.

When it comes to the natural way of life, you can take care of yourself in so many ways that you never before realized. You don't need to turn to the conventional medication with all its side effects every time you have a headache. In fact, with the use of homemade salves, creams, sprays, and tea you can take care of yourself without ever needing to worry about side effects.

If this sounds like you, you have come to the right place. In this book, you are going to discover the natural way of life, and why that is so much better than anything a doctor could give you. After all, we know what using herbs will do over the long term, but there is still little research to support what happens when you use synthetic pills over the course of years.

With this book, you are going to unlock the secret to taking care of yourself the natural way, and you are going to discover that you really can feel better than ever, you can get rid of the painful symptoms you have been feeling, and you can take care of yourself without ever needing to turn to a single synthetic pill.

This book is going to change your life for the better, and all you have to do is mix a few natural ingredients together, and you will feel great.

Keep an open mind, and you will see for yourself why you should go for the natural way of doing things.

Let's get started.

Chapter 1 – Why Go Natural?

In the world we live in, we are taught to think that conventional medication is superior to the natural medication. We are told that since it has been developed in a lab, that it is going to do a better job treating ailments than the things that have been growing in the wild.

We are taught that if anything ever hurts on us, we are to reach for a bottle of pills, and that will do the trick. We are taught never to question whether that truly is the best way of doing things.

The truth about natural medicine is that it really is highly effective, and it is still widely used around the entire world.

Many people don't agree with the use of natural medicine simply because they do not understand what it is. They assume that it is some form of not taking your body seriously, and that by going with the natural way of doing things, you aren't going to get the same level of benefits that you would get if you were to go with the conventional standards.

However, if you are serious about natural medicine, you know that you are taking your body seriously, and you are looking for something that is going to give you the results that you want.

Natural medicine, when it is done properly, is every bit as effective as using conventional medicine, but the key is to do it properly. When you are using natural medicine, you must give it time to work, and you must use it consistently so it has the time to build up in your system.

You can't expect it to work exactly like conventional medicine because it isn't going to. No matter what your expectations are, you are going to find that the natural route is going to be effective, but you have to be willing to give it a fair chance to work in your system.

On the other hand, you are going to spare your body all the harm from side effects that are listed on the side of the bottle. Sure, you might find that your headache is gone, but you are doing so at the cost of your liver. You might find that you are able to sleep better through the night, but you are doing so at the cost of your natural sleep cycle.

However, when you go the natural route, you aren't harming your body in other ways. In fact, many of the herbs are going to be so beneficial for your body that it doesn't matter why you were taking them in the first place, you are going to receive all over benefit that is greater than anything you could get from a little pill.

I encourage you to approach the concept of natural medicine with an open mind, and that you realize you are going to have to put work into it in order to reap the benefits.

Make the different recipes, use them often, and you will see your life become healthier and healthier. You are going to save money, you are going to have a greater sense of well-being, and you are going to have more energy throughout the day.

When you go natural, you do so many good things for your body that you aren't going to believe the results.

So what are you waiting for? You deserve to live the healthiest life possible, and with these all natural creams, sprays, and teas – you are going to do that very thing.

Give your body the gift of health.

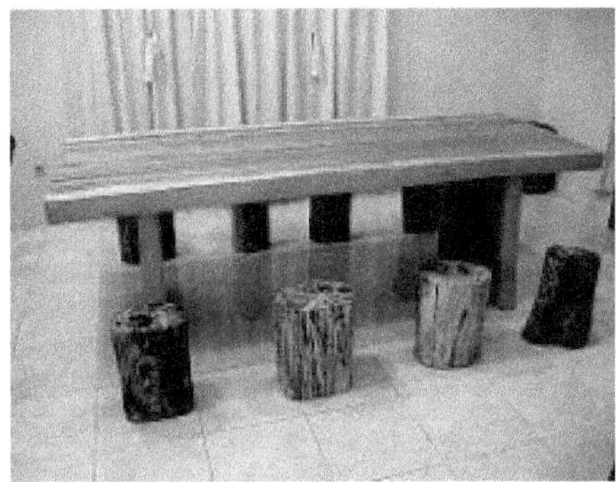

Chapter 2 – The Soothing Creams

These creams are excellent options for a variety of aches and pains. Whether you are dealing with anxiety or you are tired after a long day at work, they'll give you the relief you've been looking for.

These recipes are the perfect solution for all of the following symptoms:

- **Headaches**

- **Muscle tension**

- **PMS symptoms**

- **Arthritis pain**

- **Joint pain**

- **Anxiety**

- **Back pain**

- **Fibromyalgia**

- **Migraines**

- **Aches and pains due to the flu**

- **Residual muscle pain from a past injury**

And don't be afraid to turn to them for any other symptom you are feeling.

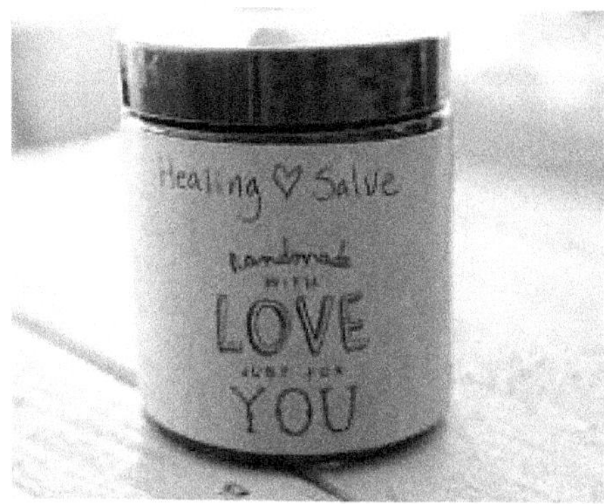

Relief Oasis

What you will need:

12 drops grapefruit oil

8 drops sunflower essential oil

½ cup coconut oil

2 tablespoons shea butter

2 teaspoons camphor crystals

Directions:

Using a double boiler or a pot converted into a double boiler, melt the shea butter until smooth. Stir in the coconut oil and camphor crystals, and once smooth add in the oils.

Transfer to an airtight container and keep ready for when aches and pains strike.

To Use:

Massage cream into the affected area and allow to sit for a few moments. The cream will begin to work quickly, and since it is used topically, it can be reapplied as often as necessary.

Use every time you feel symptoms appear.

Nothing's Better

What you will need:

8 drops tea tree oil

4 drops clove oil

½ cup coconut oil

2 tablespoons shea butter

2 teaspoons camphor crystals

Directions:

Using a double boiler or a pot converted into a double boiler, melt the shea butter until smooth. Stir in the coconut oil and camphor crystals, and once smooth add in the oils.

Transfer to an airtight container and keep ready for when aches and pains strike.

To Use:

Massage cream into the affected area and allow to sit for a few moments. The cream will begin to work quickly, and since it is used topically, it can be reapplied as often as necessary.

Use every time you feel symptoms appear.

Sweet Cream

What you will need:

15 drops rose oil

5 drops lavender oil

½ cup coconut oil

2 tablespoons shea butter

2 teaspoons camphor crystals

Directions:

Using a double boiler or a pot converted into a double boiler, melt the shea butter until smooth. Stir in the coconut oil and camphor crystals, and once smooth add in the oils.

Transfer to an airtight container and keep ready for when aches and pains strike.

To Use:

Massage cream into the affected area and allow to sit for a few moments. The cream will begin to work quickly, and since it is used topically, it can be reapplied as often as necessary.

Use every time you feel symptoms appear.

Move Again

What you will need:

12 drops frankincense oil

8 drops jasmine oil

½ cup coconut oil

2 tablespoons shea butter

2 teaspoons camphor crystals

Directions:

Using a double boiler or a pot converted into a double boiler, melt the shea butter until smooth. Stir in the coconut oil and camphor crystals, and once smooth add in the oils.

Transfer to an airtight container and keep ready for when aches and pains strike.

To Use:

Massage cream into the affected area and allow to sit for a few moments. The cream will begin to work quickly, and since it is used topically, it can be reapplied as often as necessary.

Use every time you feel symptoms appear.

Get Up and Go
What you will need:

12 drops lavender oil

12 drops lemon oil

½ cup coconut oil

2 tablespoons shea butter

2 teaspoons camphor crystals

Directions:

Using a double boiler or a pot converted into a double boiler, melt the shea butter until smooth. Stir in the coconut oil and camphor crystals, and once smooth add in the oils.

Transfer to an airtight container and keep ready for when aches and pains strike.

To Use:

Massage cream into the affected area and allow to sit for a few moments. The cream will begin to work quickly, and since it is used topically, it can be reapplied as often as necessary.

Use every time you feel symptoms appear.

Pain Be Gone
What you will need:

12 drops bergamot oil

8 drops basil oil

½ cup coconut oil

2 tablespoons shea butter

2 teaspoons camphor crystals

Directions:

Using a double boiler or a pot converted into a double boiler, melt the shea butter until smooth. Stir in the coconut oil and camphor crystals, and once smooth add in the oils.

Transfer to an airtight container and keep ready for when aches and pains strike.

To Use:

Massage cream into the affected area and allow to sit for a few moments. The cream will begin to work quickly, and since it is used topically, it can be reapplied as often as necessary.

Use every time you feel symptoms appear.

When the Cramps Strike

What you will need:

12 drops lavender oil

8 drops myrrh oil

½ cup coconut oil

2 tablespoons shea butter

2 teaspoons camphor crystals

Directions:

Using a double boiler or a pot converted into a double boiler, melt the shea butter until smooth. Stir in the coconut oil and camphor crystals, and once smooth add in the oils.

Transfer to an airtight container and keep ready for when aches and pains strike.

To Use:

Massage cream into the affected area and allow to sit for a few moments. The cream will begin to work quickly, and since it is used topically, it can be reapplied as often as necessary.

Use every time you feel symptoms appear.

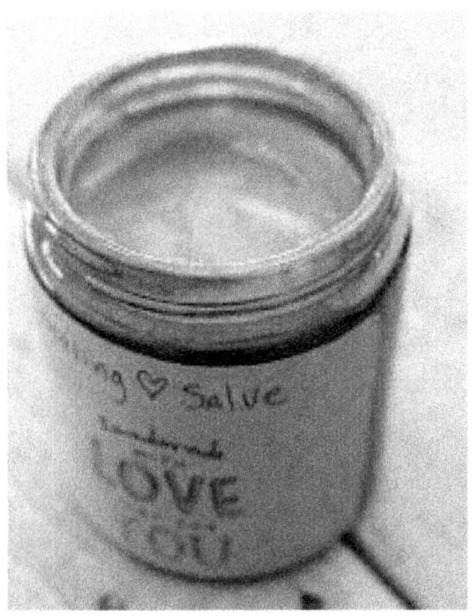

Super Cream

What you will need:

8 drops spearmint oil

8 drops peppermint oil

½ cup coconut oil

2 tablespoons shea butter

2 teaspoons camphor crystals

Directions:

Using a double boiler or a pot converted into a double boiler, melt the shea butter until smooth. Stir in the coconut oil and camphor crystals, and once smooth add in the oils.

Transfer to an airtight container and keep ready for when aches and pains strike.

To Use:

Massage cream into the affected area and allow to sit for a few moments. The cream will begin to work quickly, and since it is used topically, it can be reapplied as often as necessary.

Use every time you feel symptoms appear.

Mother's Choice
What you will need:

8 drops ginger oil

4 drops cinnamon oil

½ cup coconut oil

2 tablespoons shea butter

2 teaspoons camphor crystals

Directions:

Using a double boiler or a pot converted into a double boiler, melt the shea butter until smooth. Stir in the coconut oil and camphor crystals, and once smooth add in the oils.

Transfer to an airtight container and keep ready for when aches and pains strike.

To Use:

Massage cream into the affected area and allow to sit for a few moments. The cream will begin to work quickly, and since it is used topically, it can be reapplied as often as necessary.

Use every time you feel symptoms appear.

Now That's Relief
What you will need:

12 drops vetiver oil

3 drops helichrysum oil

½ cup coconut oil

2 tablespoons shea butter

2 teaspoons camphor crystals

Directions:

Using a double boiler or a pot converted into a double boiler, melt the shea butter until smooth. Stir in the coconut oil and camphor crystals, and once smooth add in the oils.

Transfer to an airtight container and keep ready for when aches and pains strike.

To Use:

Massage cream into the affected area and allow to sit for a few moments. The cream will begin to work quickly, and since it is used topically, it can be reapplied as often as necessary.

Use every time you feel symptoms appear.

Chapter 3 – Super Sprays

Aches and pains can strike at any time, and when they do, you want real relief – and fast. These recipes are the perfect solution for all of the following symptoms:

- **Headaches**

- **Muscle tension**

- **PMS symptoms**

- **Arthritis pain**

- **Joint pain**

- **Anxiety**

- **Back pain**

- **Fibromyalgia**

- **Migraines**

- **Muscle cramps**

If you are tired of having to cringe every time you move, or having to deal with the aches and pains deep in your muscles, try any and all of these sprays. They will be sure to do the trick, and get you up and moving in no time.

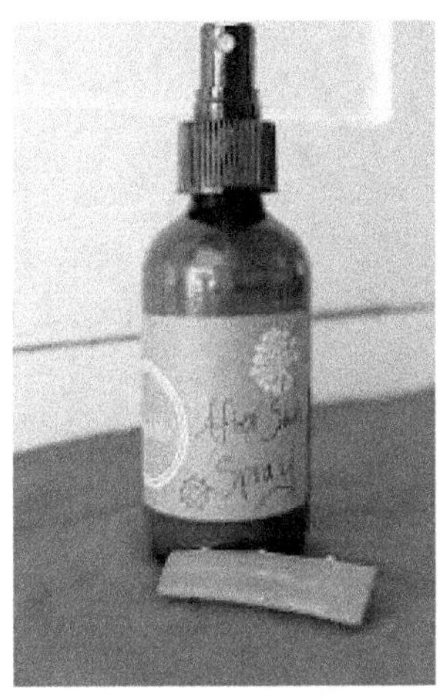

Joint Juice

What you will need:

12 drops juniper berry oil

8 drops vetiver oil

2 drops helichrysum

1 teaspoon fractionated coconut oil

Enough magnesium oil to fill your bottle after adding the first ingredients

Small spray bottle

Directions:

Combine all ingredients in a small spray bottle, and remember to shake well when you are ready to use.

To Use:

As a topical spray, you can use this any time you are feeling aches, pains, or discomfort of any kind. Simply spritz the spray over the affected area, then gently massage into your skin.

Works quickly, and can be reapplied as often as needed.

Arthritis Kicker

What you will need:

12 drops ginger oil

3 drops cinnamon oil

2 drops helichrysum

1 teaspoon fractionated coconut oil

Enough magnesium oil to fill your bottle after adding the first ingredients

Small spray bottle

Directions:

Combine all ingredients in a small spray bottle, and remember to shake well when you are ready to use.

To Use:

As a topical spray, you can use this any time you are feeling aches, pains, or discomfort of any kind. Simply spritz the spray over the affected area, then gently massage into your skin.

Works quickly, and can be reapplied as often as needed.

Real Relief

What you will need:

12 drops grapefruit oil

6 drops geranium oil

2 drops helichrysum

1 teaspoon fractionated coconut oil

Enough magnesium oil to fill your bottle after adding the first ingredients

Small spray bottle

Directions:

Combine all ingredients in a small spray bottle, and remember to shake well when you are ready to use.

To Use:

As a topical spray, you can use this any time you are feeling aches, pains, or discomfort of any kind. Simply spritz the spray over the affected area, then gently massage into your skin.

Works quickly, and can be reapplied as often as needed.

Painstakingly Awesome

What you will need:

6 drops chamomile oil

6 drops jojoba oil

2 drops helichrysum

1 teaspoon fractionated coconut oil

Enough magnesium oil to fill your bottle after adding the first ingredients

Small spray bottle

Directions:

Combine all ingredients in a small spray bottle, and remember to shake well when you are ready to use.

To Use:

As a topical spray, you can use this any time you are feeling aches, pains, or discomfort of any kind. Simply spritz the spray over the affected area, then gently massage into your skin.

Works quickly, and can be reapplied as often as needed.

Back in a Flash

What you will need:

8 drops bergamot oil

2 drops ylang ylang oil

2 drops helichrysum

1 teaspoon fractionated coconut oil

Enough magnesium oil to fill your bottle after adding the first ingredients

Small spray bottle

Directions:

Combine all ingredients in a small spray bottle, and remember to shake well when you are ready to use.

To Use:

As a topical spray, you can use this any time you are feeling aches, pains, or discomfort of any kind. Simply spritz the spray over the affected area, then gently massage into your skin.

Works quickly, and can be reapplied as often as needed.

Sonic Spray

What you will need:

8 drops clary sage oil

4 drops garlic oil

2 drops helichrysum

1 teaspoon fractionated coconut oil

Enough magnesium oil to fill your bottle after adding the first ingredients

Small spray bottle

Directions:

Combine all ingredients in a small spray bottle, and remember to shake well when you are ready to use.

To Use:

As a topical spray, you can use this any time you are feeling aches, pains, or discomfort of any kind. Simply spritz the spray over the affected area, then gently massage into your skin.

Works quickly, and can be reapplied as often as needed.

Healthy Healing

What you will need:

8 drops peppermint oil

2 drops tea tree oil

2 drops helichrysum

1 teaspoon fractionated coconut oil

Enough magnesium oil to fill your bottle after adding the first ingredients

Small spray bottle

Directions:

Combine all ingredients in a small spray bottle, and remember to shake well when you are ready to use.

To Use:

As a topical spray, you can use this any time you are feeling aches, pains, or discomfort of any kind. Simply spritz the spray over the affected area, then gently massage into your skin.

Works quickly, and can be reapplied as often as needed.

Healing Breeze

What you will need:

12 drops frankincense oil

4 drops lavender oil

2 drops helichrysum

1 teaspoon fractionated coconut oil

Enough magnesium oil to fill your bottle after adding the first ingredients

Small spray bottle

Directions:

Combine all ingredients in a small spray bottle, and remember to shake well when you are ready to use.

To Use:

As a topical spray, you can use this any time you are feeling aches, pains, or discomfort of any kind. Simply spritz the spray over the affected area, then gently massage into your skin.

Works quickly, and can be reapplied as often as needed.

Feeling Fresh

What you will need:

7 drops eucalyptus oil

3 drops peppermint oil

2 drops helichrysum

1 teaspoon fractionated coconut oil

Enough magnesium oil to fill your bottle after adding the first ingredients

Small spray bottle

Directions:

Combine all ingredients in a small spray bottle, and remember to shake well when you are ready to use.

To Use:

As a topical spray, you can use this any time you are feeling aches, pains, or discomfort of any kind. Simply spritz the spray over the affected area, then gently massage into your skin.

Works quickly, and can be reapplied as often as needed.

All Better

What you will need:

8 drops peppermint oil

2 drops geranium oil

2 drops helichrysum

1 teaspoon fractionated coconut oil

Enough magnesium oil to fill your bottle after adding the first ingredients

Small spray bottle

Directions:

Combine all ingredients in a small spray bottle, and remember to shake well when you are ready to use.

To Use:

As a topical spray, you can use this any time you are feeling aches, pains, or discomfort of any kind. Simply spritz the spray over the affected area, then gently massage into your skin.

Works quickly, and can be reapplied as often as needed.

Chapter 4 – From the Inside Out: Pain Relieving Teas

Tea is an excellent way to heal your body from the inside out. Not only can you use it to soothe an upset stomach or sore throat, but you can use it to alleviate stress or anxiety, too.

Try these herbs next time you are feeling any of the following symptoms, and you are going to be back to your old self in no time.

These teas are perfect for:

- **Stress relief**

- **Anxiety relief**

- **Stomach aches**

- **Headaches**

- **Migraines**

- **Joint pain**

- **Muscle pain**

- **Sore throat**

- **Cold and flu symptoms**

Instead of reaching for a bottle of pills, next time opt for a glass of herbal tea, and watch the health benefits comes rolling back in.

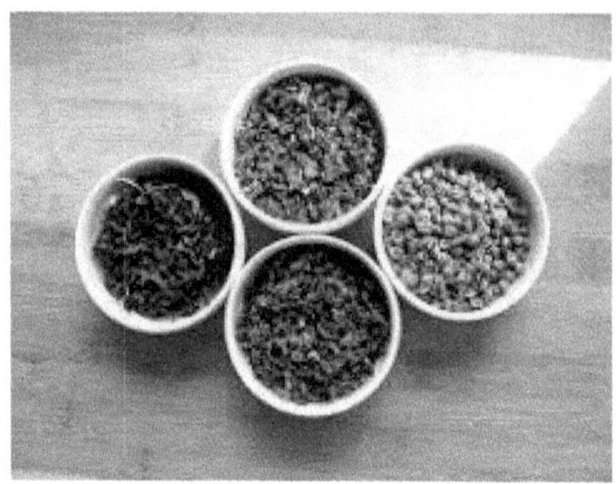

Sore Throat Soother

What you will need:

1 teaspoon white willow bark

1 teaspoon crushed, dried blueberries

1 tablespoon black tea leaves

1 packet stevia

Directions:

Place all the herbs in a tea ball and allow to steep for 5 minutes in almost boiling water. Allow the water to cool enough to safely drink, and enjoy.

To Use:

Brew a cup and sip on it every time you feel symptoms. Since you are ingesting these herbs, it is best to limit yourself to 2 or 3 cups per day. Continue as long as symptoms persist.

The Stomach Settler

What you will need:

1 teaspoon dried ginger

1 teaspoon rosemary leaves

1 tablespoon black tea leaves

1 packet stevia

Directions:

Place all the herbs in a tea ball and allow to steep for 5 minutes in almost boiling water. Allow the water to cool enough to safely drink, and enjoy.

To Use:

Brew a cup and sip on it every time you feel symptoms. Since you are ingesting these herbs, it is best to limit yourself to 2 or 3 cups per day. Continue as long as symptoms persist.

Stress Be Gone

What you will need:

1 teaspoon lavender leaves

1 teaspoon lemon zest

1 tablespoon black tea leaves

1 packet stevia

Directions:

Place all the herbs in a tea ball and allow to steep for 5 minutes in almost boiling water. Allow the water to cool enough to safely drink, and enjoy.

To Use:

Brew a cup and sip on it every time you feel symptoms. Since you are ingesting these herbs, it is best to limit yourself to 2 or 3 cups per day. Continue as long as symptoms persist.

Cold Kicker

What you will need:

1 teaspoon peppermint leaves

1 teaspoon cinnamon

1 tablespoon black tea leaves

1 packet stevia

Directions:

Place all the herbs in a tea ball and allow to steep for 5 minutes in almost boiling water. Allow the water to cool enough to safely drink, and enjoy.

To Use:

Brew a cup and sip on it every time you feel symptoms. Since you are ingesting these herbs, it is best to limit yourself to 2 or 3 cups per day. Continue as long as symptoms persist.

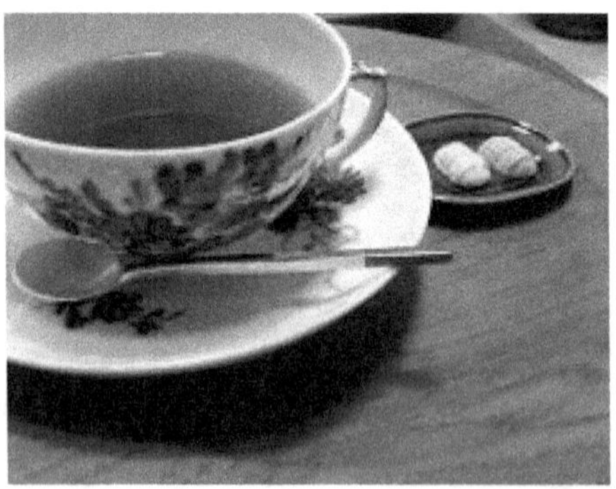

Nature's Kiss
What you will need:

1 teaspoon cloves

1 teaspoon garlic

1 tablespoon black tea leaves

1 packet stevia

Directions:

Place all the herbs in a tea ball and allow to steep for 5 minutes in almost boiling water. Allow the water to cool enough to safely drink, and enjoy.

To Use:

Brew a cup and sip on it every time you feel symptoms. Since you are ingesting these herbs, it is best to limit yourself to 2 or 3 cups per day. Continue as long as symptoms persist.

No Worries
What you will need:

1 teaspoon peppermint leaves

1 teaspoon dried ginger

1 tablespoon black tea leaves

1 packet stevia

Directions:

Place all the herbs in a tea ball and allow to steep for 5 minutes in almost boiling water. Allow the water to cool enough to safely drink, and enjoy.

To Use:

Brew a cup and sip on it every time you feel symptoms. Since you are ingesting these herbs, it is best to limit yourself to 2 or 3 cups per day. Continue as long as symptoms persist.

Sleep Well

What you will need:

1 teaspoon peppermint leaves

1 teaspoon lavender leaves

1 tablespoon black tea leaves

1 packet stevia

Directions:

Place all the herbs in a tea ball and allow to steep for 5 minutes in almost boiling water. Allow the water to cool enough to safely drink, and enjoy.

To Use:

Brew a cup and sip on it every time you feel symptoms. Since you are ingesting these herbs, it is best to limit yourself to 2 or 3 cups per day. Continue as long as symptoms persist.

Wellness Tea

What you will need:

1 tablespoon dried, crushed cherries

1 teaspoon cinnamon

1 tablespoon black tea leaves

1 packet stevia

Directions:

Place all the herbs in a tea ball and allow to steep for 5 minutes in almost boiling water. Allow the water to cool enough to safely drink, and enjoy.

To Use:

Brew a cup and sip on it every time you feel symptoms. Since you are ingesting these herbs, it is best to limit yourself to 2 or 3 cups per day. Continue as long as symptoms persist.

More Than Tea
What you will need:

1 teaspoon cinnamon

1 teaspoon ginger

1 tablespoon black tea leaves

1 packet stevia

Directions:

Place all the herbs in a tea ball and allow to steep for 5 minutes in almost boiling water. Allow the water to cool enough to safely drink, and enjoy.

To Use:

Brew a cup and sip on it every time you feel symptoms. Since you are ingesting these herbs, it is best to limit yourself to 2 or 3 cups per day. Continue as long as symptoms persist.

Doctor's Helper
What you will need:

1 teaspoon turmeric powder

1 teaspoon ground ginger

Pinch of black pepper

1 tablespoon black tea leaves

1 packet stevia

Directions:

Place all the herbs in a tea ball and allow to steep for 5 minutes in almost boiling water. Allow the water to cool enough to safely drink, and enjoy.

To Use:

Brew a cup and sip on it every time you feel symptoms. Since you are ingesting these herbs, it is best to limit yourself to 2 or 3 cups per day. Continue as long as symptoms persist.

Conclusion

There you have it, everything you need to know to use herbs, homemade sprays, and homemade creams to take care of any aches and pains that come your way. Though we are often told that we must use the modern remedies that are available in the store, the fact of the matter is that you can heal yourself using entirely natural ingredients whenever you wish.

I hope this book inspires you to take your health to the next level, and that you take what you have learned here and apply it to your healthcare regimen. From now on, whenever you feel like you're getting sick, whenever you have a headache or a migraine, or whenever you have a scrape or a cut that you want to go away, you have a natural remedy to use.

I know this book is going to change the way you view medication and the natural world, and it's going to give you more rich health benefits than you ever thought possible. You are going to fall in love with each of these recipes, and you are going to fall in love with the results.

You will be saved the headache of side effects, you will save money, and you will do yourself a favor beyond what you ever thought possible.

Happy healing.

FREE Bonus Reminder

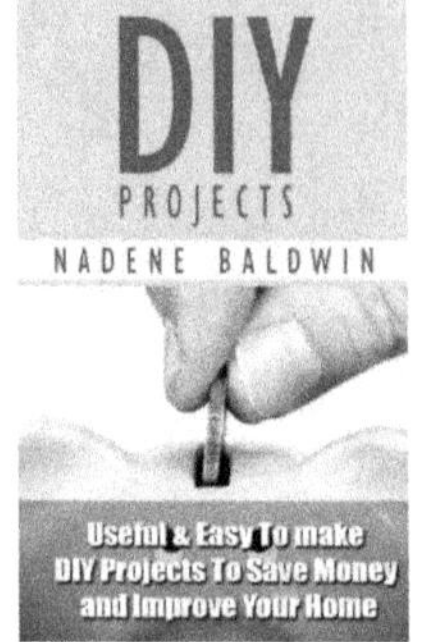

If you have not grabbed it yet, please go ahead and download your special bonus report *"DIY Projects. 13 Useful & Easy To Make DIY Projects To Save Money & Improve Your Home!"*
Simply Click the Button Below

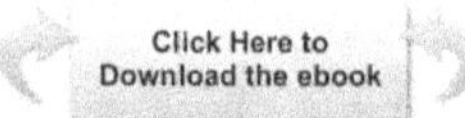

OR **Go to This Page**
http://diyhomecraft.com/free

BONUS #2: More Free & Discounted Books or Products
Do you want to receive more Free/Discounted Books or Products?
We have a mailing list where we send out our new Books or Products when they go free or with a discount on Amazon. Click on the link below to sign up for Free & Discount Book & Product Promotions.
=> Sign Up for Free & Discount Book & Product Promotions <=

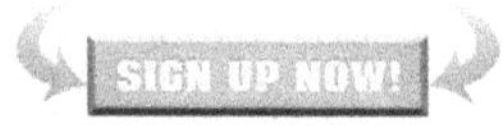

OR Go to this URL
http://bit.ly/1WBb1Ek